The Ethical Hacker: Unraveling Technology Dilemmas for Student Coders

AF571119

Natalia Ivanova

Copyright © [2023]

Title: The Ethical Hacker: Unraveling Technology Dilemmas for Student Coders

Author's: Natalia Ivanova.

All rights reserved. No part of this publication may be reproduced, stored in a retrieval system, or transmitted in any form or by any means, electronic, mechanical, photocopying, recording, or otherwise, without the prior written permission of the publisher or author, except in the case of brief quotations embodied in critical reviews and certain other non-commercial uses permitted by copyright law.

This book was printed and published by [Publisher's: Natalia Ivanova] in [2023]

ISBN:

TABLE OF CONTENTS

Chapter 1: Introduction to Technology Ethics

Understanding the Importance of Technology Ethics

In today's digital age, technology plays a vital role in almost every aspect of our lives. From communication and education to healthcare and entertainment, technology has revolutionized the way we live and work. However, just like any other tool, it can be used for both positive and negative purposes. This is where the importance of technology ethics comes into play.

Technology ethics refers to the moral principles and guidelines that govern the use of technology. It involves understanding the impact of technology on individuals, society, and the environment, and making responsible choices that align with ethical values. As students and future coders, it is crucial to grasp the significance of technology ethics and integrate it into our work and decision-making processes.

One of the primary reasons why technology ethics is essential is because it helps protect individuals' privacy and security. In today's interconnected world, the collection and use of personal data have become widespread. Ethical considerations ensure that individuals' information is handled with care, and their privacy is respected. By adhering to ethical practices, we can prevent unauthorized access, data breaches, and other cybercrimes that compromise people's sensitive information.

Furthermore, technology ethics helps promote fairness and equality. As the digital divide widens, it is crucial to ensure that everyone has equal access to technology and its benefits. Ethical considerations help prevent discrimination and bias in the development and deployment of technology. By designing inclusive and accessible technologies, we can bridge the gap between different socio-economic backgrounds and create a more equitable society.

Additionally, technology ethics encourages sustainability and environmental responsibility. The production and disposal of technology have significant environmental impacts. Ethical practices prioritize the use of eco-friendly materials, energy-efficient designs, and responsible e-waste management. By considering the environmental consequences of our technological choices, we can minimize our carbon footprint and contribute to a greener future.

Moreover, technology ethics fosters transparency and accountability. As creators and users of technology, it is important to understand the potential consequences of our actions. Ethical considerations help us take responsibility for the outcomes of our technological advancements. By being transparent about the intentions and potential risks associated with technology, we can build trust among users and ensure that our innovations serve the greater good.

In conclusion, understanding the importance of technology ethics is crucial for students in the field of coding. By integrating ethical considerations into our work, we can protect individuals' privacy, promote fairness and equality, encourage sustainability, and foster transparency and accountability. As future coders, it is our responsibility to use technology ethically and contribute to a more ethical and inclusive digital society.

Ethical Considerations in the Digital Age

In our increasingly interconnected world, the digital age has brought about numerous advancements and opportunities. However, along with these progressions, there are also ethical considerations that need to be addressed. As student coders, it is essential to understand and navigate these ethical dilemmas to ensure that our work aligns with ethical standards and principles. This subchapter aims to shed light on the ethical considerations that arise in the digital age and provides guidance on how to approach them.

One of the prominent ethical considerations in the digital age is privacy. With the vast amount of data being collected and shared online, it is crucial to respect individuals' privacy rights. As student coders, we must be mindful of the data we collect, store, and use, ensuring that it is done with proper consent and within legal boundaries. Additionally, we should be wary of the potential for data breaches and take necessary precautions to protect sensitive information.

Another ethical dilemma is cybersecurity. As we develop coding skills, it is essential to recognize the potential harm that can arise from our work if it falls into the wrong hands. We must prioritize cybersecurity measures and strive to create systems that are secure and resilient against potential threats. This includes understanding and adhering to ethical hacking practices, ensuring that our work is not used for malicious purposes.

The digital age also presents challenges related to intellectual property. As student coders, it is crucial to respect copyright laws and intellectual property rights. We should refrain from plagiarizing or using others' work without proper attribution. This includes open-source projects, where it is essential to understand and comply with the licensing terms and conditions.

Moreover, the digital age brings forth concerns regarding digital divide and accessibility. As student coders, we have a responsibility to create inclusive and accessible technology solutions that cater to diverse populations. This means considering factors such as usability, affordability, and availability for individuals with disabilities or limited access to resources.

Lastly, ethical considerations in the digital age extend to the impact of technology on society. As student coders, we should be aware of the potential consequences of our work on individuals, communities, and the environment. We must strive to develop technologies that promote fairness, social responsibility, and sustainability.

In conclusion, the digital age presents an array of ethical considerations that student coders must be cognizant of. By understanding and addressing these dilemmas, we can ensure that our work aligns with ethical principles and contributes positively to society. By promoting privacy, prioritizing cybersecurity, respecting intellectual property, fostering inclusivity, and considering the societal impact, we can navigate the digital age ethically and responsibly.

The Role of Ethical Hackers in Technology

In today's rapidly evolving digital landscape, the role of ethical hackers has become increasingly crucial. As students venturing into the world of coding and technology, it is imperative to understand the significance and ethical implications of the work carried out by these individuals. This subchapter aims to shed light on the role of ethical hackers in technology, emphasizing the importance of ethics in this field.

Ethical hackers, also known as white hat hackers, are computer security experts who specialize in identifying vulnerabilities and weaknesses in computer systems, networks, and software. Their main objective is to uncover potential security flaws before malicious hackers can exploit them. By simulating real-world cyber-attacks, ethical hackers help organizations and individuals protect their digital assets and maintain the integrity of their systems.

One of the key aspects that differentiate ethical hackers from their malicious counterparts is their adherence to a strict code of ethics. Ethical hackers must operate within legal boundaries, seeking explicit permission from the owners of the systems they are testing. They are bound by a set of ethical guidelines that prioritize privacy, consent, and responsible disclosure of vulnerabilities. By upholding these principles, ethical hackers ensure that their actions contribute to the overall security and well-being of the digital ecosystem.

Ethics play a vital role in the work of ethical hackers. They must navigate complex moral dilemmas, balancing the need to uncover vulnerabilities with the responsibility to protect user privacy and data.

Additionally, they must carefully consider the potential consequences of their actions, ensuring that the information they uncover is used solely for the purpose of improving security measures.

For students interested in pursuing a career in ethical hacking or cybersecurity, a strong foundation in ethics is essential. It is not enough to possess technical skills; one must also develop a deep understanding of the ethical implications of their work. By adhering to a strong ethical framework, students can ensure that they contribute positively to the advancement of technology while maintaining the highest standards of integrity.

In conclusion, the role of ethical hackers in technology cannot be understated. Their work is instrumental in safeguarding digital systems and protecting against cyber threats. As students exploring the world of coding and technology, it is crucial to recognize the importance of ethics in this field. By upholding ethical principles and understanding the implications of their actions, students can become responsible and effective ethical hackers, contributing to the betterment of cybersecurity and technology as a whole.

Chapter 2: The Fundamentals of Ethical Hacking

Defining Ethical Hacking

In today's digital age, where technology has become an integral part of our lives, the concept of ethical hacking has gained significant importance. As students venturing into the world of coding, it is essential for us to understand what ethical hacking truly means and how it aligns with the principles of ethics.

Ethical hacking, also known as white-hat hacking or penetration testing, refers to the practice of testing computer systems, networks, or applications with the permission of the owner to identify security vulnerabilities. The goal of ethical hacking is to improve the overall security of these systems by identifying weaknesses before malicious hackers can exploit them.

Unlike the malicious activities associated with hacking, ethical hacking is carried out by individuals with a deep understanding of computer systems and security protocols. These ethical hackers, or security professionals, use their skills and knowledge to assess the security posture of organizations, identify vulnerabilities, and provide solutions to strengthen their defenses.

However, ethical hacking is not just about technical skills. It is also deeply rooted in the principles of ethics. Ethical hackers must adhere to a strict code of conduct, which includes obtaining proper authorization before conducting any tests, respecting privacy and confidentiality, and ensuring that their actions do not cause harm or disruption to the systems they are testing.

Ethics play a crucial role in guiding the actions of ethical hackers. They must always prioritize the well-being and safety of individuals and organizations, ensuring that their testing activities do not compromise the privacy or integrity of sensitive data. Ethical hackers are also committed to continuous learning and staying up-to-date with the latest security trends and technologies, as this knowledge is essential to effectively protect against evolving threats.

For students interested in pursuing a career in ethical hacking, it is important to understand the significance of ethics in this field. Ethical hacking provides a unique opportunity to use our coding skills for the greater good, helping organizations identify and mitigate vulnerabilities before they can be exploited by malicious actors. By following ethical guidelines and principles, we can contribute to creating a safer digital space for all.

In conclusion, ethical hacking is a discipline that combines technical expertise with ethical principles to identify and address security vulnerabilities. As students, we have the responsibility to approach ethical hacking with integrity, professionalism, and a commitment to making a positive impact on the digital world.

Ethical Hacking Methodologies

Ethical hacking is an essential skill that every student interested in technology and coding should be familiar with. In this subchapter, we will explore the methodologies and frameworks that ethical hackers use to ensure their actions are within the boundaries of ethics and legality.

Ethical hacking, also known as white-hat hacking, refers to the practice of identifying vulnerabilities and weaknesses in computer systems, networks, and applications. The ultimate goal is to protect these systems from malicious attacks and unauthorized access. However, it is crucial to conduct ethical hacking in an ethical and responsible manner, respecting the privacy and rights of others.

One popular methodology used by ethical hackers is the "Open Source Security Testing Methodology Manual" (OSSTMM). This framework provides a comprehensive approach to assessing security risks and vulnerabilities. It covers areas such as information security, physical security, operations security, and telecommunications security. By following the OSSTMM, ethical hackers can ensure a systematic and thorough examination of potential vulnerabilities.

Another methodology widely used is the "Penetration Testing Execution Standard" (PTES). This framework guides ethical hackers through the entire process of penetration testing, from initial planning to reporting and remediation. PTES emphasizes the importance of obtaining proper authorization, maintaining strict confidentiality, and documenting every step of the testing process.

When conducting ethical hacking, it is essential to follow a code of ethics. Organizations such as the International Council of Electronic Commerce Consultants (EC-Council) have established ethical guidelines for ethical hackers. These guidelines emphasize the importance of obtaining proper consent, respecting privacy, and protecting sensitive information.

Moreover, ethical hackers should always prioritize the confidentiality, integrity, and availability of the systems they are testing. They must also be transparent in their communication with the organization they are working for, providing regular updates, and sharing findings responsibly.

Ethics plays a significant role in ethical hacking, as it ensures that the practice remains legitimate and beneficial. As students of technology and coding, it is essential to understand the ethical implications of hacking and adhere to ethical standards. By doing so, we can contribute to the development of secure systems and protect against potential threats.

In conclusion, ethical hacking methodologies provide a structured approach to identifying vulnerabilities and ensuring the security of computer systems and networks. By following frameworks like OSSTMM and PTES, and adhering to ethical guidelines, student coders can develop their skills in an ethical and responsible manner. Understanding the importance of ethics in ethical hacking is crucial for the development of a secure and trustworthy digital landscape.

Ethical Hacking Tools and Techniques

In today's digital age, where technology is an integral part of our lives, the need for ethical hackers has become paramount. As students with a keen interest in coding and a strong commitment to ethics, it is crucial to understand the tools and techniques employed by ethical hackers to ensure the security and integrity of computer systems.

Ethical hacking, also known as penetration testing or white-hat hacking, involves identifying vulnerabilities in computer systems and networks to strengthen their security. This subchapter aims to provide you, as student coders with an ethical mindset, an overview of the tools and techniques used by ethical hackers.

One of the fundamental tools used by ethical hackers is a vulnerability scanner. These scanners help identify potential weaknesses in a system by scanning it for known vulnerabilities and misconfigurations. Some popular vulnerability scanners include Nessus, OpenVAS, and Nexpose.

Another essential tool is the password cracking software, which helps ethical hackers determine the strength of passwords used within a system. Tools like John the Ripper and Hashcat are commonly used to crack passwords by employing various methods such as brute-force attacks, dictionary attacks, and rainbow table attacks.

Network analyzers, such as Wireshark, are vital for capturing and analyzing network traffic. Ethical hackers can use these tools to identify any potential security flaws in the network infrastructure, detect suspicious activities, and analyze packet data in real-time.

Additionally, ethical hackers rely on social engineering techniques to exploit human vulnerabilities. Techniques such as phishing, pretexting, and baiting are used to manipulate individuals into revealing sensitive information or granting unauthorized access. It is essential to understand these techniques to be able to defend against them effectively.

As student coders committed to ethics, it is essential to mention that ethical hacking should always be performed legally and with proper authorization. Ethical hackers should adhere to a code of conduct and obtain permission from the system owners before conducting any security assessments.

By learning about these ethical hacking tools and techniques, you can develop a strong foundation in cybersecurity and contribute to safeguarding digital systems. Remember, as future professionals, it is our responsibility to use our knowledge and skills ethically, ensuring a secure and trustworthy digital landscape for all.

Chapter 3: Legal and Ethical Frameworks

Laws and Regulations in Technology

In the fast-paced world of technology, it is essential for student coders to understand the importance of laws and regulations that govern their field of work. As technology continues to evolve and shape our lives, ethical considerations become increasingly crucial. In this subchapter, we will delve into the laws and regulations in technology and explore their significance for students in the coding community.

One of the fundamental aspects of technology ethics is the legal framework that guides innovation and protects individuals and society. Laws and regulations ensure that technology is developed and used responsibly, with due consideration for privacy, security, and fairness. As students entering the world of coding, understanding these laws and regulations is essential for both personal and professional growth.

Privacy laws are of particular importance in the technology sector. Students must familiarize themselves with regulations such as the General Data Protection Regulation (GDPR) and the California Consumer Privacy Act (CCPA). These laws outline the rights and responsibilities of companies and individuals when it comes to collecting, storing, and processing personal data. By adhering to these regulations, student coders can ensure that they build ethical and responsible systems that protect user privacy.

Intellectual property laws are another crucial aspect of technology ethics. Students must understand copyright, trademark, and patent laws to respect and protect the intellectual property of others. By obtaining proper licenses and permissions, coders can avoid legal disputes and foster an environment of innovation and collaboration.

Additionally, laws and regulations related to cybersecurity play a vital role in the technology industry. Students should be knowledgeable about laws that address hacking, data breaches, and cybercrime. By understanding these regulations, coders can develop secure systems and protect their users from potential threats.

Furthermore, ethical considerations in technology extend beyond legal obligations. Students should be aware of ethical frameworks and principles that guide their decision-making process. The subchapter will explore concepts such as ethical hacking, responsible disclosure, and the importance of transparency in technology development.

By understanding and complying with laws and regulations in technology, student coders can contribute to a more ethical and responsible technological landscape. This subchapter aims to equip students with the necessary knowledge to navigate the legal and ethical challenges they may encounter in their coding journey. With a strong foundation in laws and regulations, students can become ethical hackers who unravel technology dilemmas while upholding the principles of integrity, privacy, and fairness.

Ethical Guidelines for Ethical Hackers

In the dynamic world of technology, where cyber threats are becoming increasingly sophisticated, the need for ethical hackers has never been greater. Ethical hackers, also known as white hat hackers, play a crucial role in safeguarding our digital ecosystems while adhering to a strong set of ethical guidelines. This subchapter aims to outline the important ethical considerations that student coders should take into account when embarking on a career in ethical hacking.

1. Obtain Proper Authorization: Ethical hackers must always seek permission from the appropriate parties before conducting any security assessments or penetration testing. Without proper authorization, even the most well-intentioned actions can be considered illegal and unethical.

2. Respect Data Privacy: The ethical hacker must prioritize the privacy and confidentiality of any data they encounter during their assessments. It is essential to handle sensitive information responsibly, ensuring it is not misused, disclosed, or accessed by unauthorized individuals.

3. Maintain Integrity: Ethical hackers should always act with integrity, honesty, and transparency. It is important to accurately report findings and vulnerabilities discovered during assessments, without exaggeration or manipulation. The focus should be on improving security, not on personal gain or reputation.

4. Continuous Learning and Professionalism: The field of ethical hacking is constantly evolving, and staying up-to-date with the latest techniques, tools, and technologies is crucial. Ethical hackers should

engage in continuous learning, pursuing certifications and professional development opportunities to enhance their skills and knowledge. Professionalism should be maintained at all times, respecting fellow professionals and collaborating effectively.

5. Be Mindful of Impact: Ethical hackers should consider the potential consequences of their actions. It is important to minimize any disruption caused during security assessments and avoid damaging systems or networks. The goal is to improve security, not cause harm.

6. Follow Legal and Regulatory Frameworks: Ethical hackers must comply with all applicable laws, regulations, and guidelines during their assessments. It is essential to be well-versed in national and international legal frameworks, ensuring that actions taken are within the boundaries of these regulations.

By adhering to these ethical guidelines, student coders can become responsible and respected ethical hackers. Remember, the ultimate goal is to protect and secure our digital infrastructure while maintaining the highest standards of ethics and professionalism. Your skills as an ethical hacker can make a significant positive impact on the world of technology, and it is your responsibility to use them wisely and ethically.

Balancing Ethics and Legal Compliance

In today's digital age, where technology continues to shape our lives and societies, it becomes increasingly important to address the ethical considerations that arise in the field of coding and cybersecurity. As aspiring student coders, it is crucial that we not only possess technical skills but also understand the ethical implications of our work. This subchapter titled "Balancing Ethics and Legal Compliance" aims to shed light on the delicate balance between ethical decision-making and legal compliance that is essential for all student coders to comprehend.

Ethics, in the context of coding, refers to the moral principles and values that guide our actions and decisions as programmers. It involves understanding the potential impacts of our code on individuals, communities, and society as a whole. As student coders, we have the responsibility to consider the ethical implications of our work, ensuring that our code does not harm or infringe upon the rights of others.

However, our ethical responsibilities must also be balanced with legal compliance. While ethical considerations may often go beyond what is strictly required by the law, it is crucial to understand and adhere to legal guidelines and regulations. By following the law, we can ensure that our actions as coders are within the legal boundaries, protecting ourselves and our work from legal repercussions.

One of the primary ethical dilemmas student coders often face is the issue of privacy. As we develop applications and software, we must consider the privacy rights of users and the potential risks associated with collecting and storing personal data. Respecting user privacy is not only an ethical obligation but also a legal requirement in many jurisdictions. By incorporating privacy-enhancing techniques and obtaining explicit user consent, we can strike a balance between ethical responsibility and legal compliance.

Another crucial ethical consideration for student coders is the concept of intellectual property. It is essential to respect the copyrights, patents, and trademarks of others, ensuring that our code does not infringe upon someone else's work. Furthermore, open-source software and collaborative development present their own ethical challenges, where we must acknowledge and respect the licenses and terms of use associated with such projects.

As student coders, we must strive to strike a balance between ethical decision-making and legal compliance. By understanding the potential impacts of our code, respecting user privacy, and acknowledging intellectual property rights, we can navigate the complex landscape of coding ethics. Ultimately, our ability to balance ethics and legal compliance will not only shape our professional careers but also contribute to a more responsible and ethical technology-driven world.

Chapter 4: Privacy and Data Protection

The Concept of Privacy in the Digital Era

In today's interconnected world, where technology permeates every aspect of our lives, the concept of privacy has become increasingly relevant and complex. The digital era has reshaped the way we communicate, share information, and interact with each other. As students and aspiring coders, it is crucial to delve into the ethical implications surrounding privacy in the digital age.

Privacy, traditionally understood as the right to be left alone and to have control over personal information, has taken on new dimensions in the digital era. With the proliferation of social media platforms, online shopping, and digital communication tools, our personal data is constantly being collected, analyzed, and shared. This raises questions about the boundaries between public and private, and the extent to which we can safeguard our personal information.

Ethics play a significant role in this discussion. As student coders, it is essential to recognize the ethical responsibilities associated with handling data and developing technologies. This subchapter will explore the ethical dilemmas that arise when navigating privacy concerns in the digital era.

One major dilemma is the trade-off between convenience and privacy. While digital technologies have undoubtedly made our lives easier, they often require us to disclose personal information. We willingly share our location, preferences, and even intimate details with various online platforms. Balancing the benefits of convenience with the potential risks to our privacy is a challenge we must address ethically.

Another ethical issue revolves around data breaches and cyberattacks. As student coders, we must understand the importance of securing data and developing robust systems. With the increasing frequency of high-profile hacking incidents, the need for ethical hackers to protect sensitive information has never been more critical. We will explore how ethical hacking can be employed to identify vulnerabilities and ensure the privacy of users.

Furthermore, we will delve into the ethical considerations related to surveillance and government intrusion. In the name of national security, governments around the world are implementing surveillance programs that monitor citizens' online activities. Striking a balance between security and personal privacy is an ongoing ethical debate, and as students, it is our responsibility to critically analyze these issues.

In conclusion, the concept of privacy in the digital era is multifaceted and demands ethical contemplation. As student coders, understanding the implications of privacy in the digital age is crucial for developing responsible and ethical technologies. This subchapter will explore the ethical dilemmas surrounding privacy, including the trade-off between convenience and privacy, data breaches and cyberattacks, and government surveillance. By examining these topics, we can foster a deeper understanding of the ethical challenges and make informed decisions as we navigate the ever-evolving digital landscape.

Data Protection Laws and Best Practices

In today's digital age, where personal information is constantly being collected, stored, and shared, it is crucial to understand the importance of data protection laws and best practices. As students and aspiring coders, it is essential to approach technology with an ethical mindset and respect for individual privacy. This subchapter aims to shed light on the significance of data protection laws and provide students with best practices to ensure ethical conduct in their coding endeavors.

Data protection laws are designed to safeguard the personal information of individuals and ensure its secure handling. These laws vary across countries, but they all share a common goal of protecting sensitive data from unauthorized access, use, and disclosure. Students must familiarize themselves with the data protection laws in their respective regions to ensure compliance and avoid legal consequences.

One of the fundamental principles of data protection is informed consent. As ethical coders, it is essential to obtain explicit permission from individuals before collecting their personal data. This includes explaining the purpose of data collection and providing options for individuals to control how their data is used. Transparency is key to building trust and maintaining ethical standards.

Another best practice in data protection is minimizing data collection and retention. Students should strive to collect only the necessary data required for their coding projects and avoid storing it for longer than necessary. By adopting a minimalist approach, students can reduce the potential risks associated with data breaches and unauthorized access.

Data encryption is a crucial tool in protecting personal information. Students should implement encryption techniques to secure data both at rest and in transit. Encryption ensures that even if data is intercepted or accessed without authorization, it remains unreadable and unusable to unauthorized individuals.

Regularly updating and patching software is another essential best practice to protect data. Students must stay up-to-date with the latest security patches and ensure that their coding projects are equipped with robust security measures. By keeping software updated, students can mitigate vulnerabilities that may be exploited by hackers.

Lastly, students must prioritize user privacy throughout the development process. This includes incorporating privacy-by-design principles, conducting privacy impact assessments, and regularly auditing their coding projects for potential privacy risks. By proactively considering privacy concerns, students can ensure that their coding endeavors align with ethical standards and respect individual privacy rights.

In conclusion, data protection laws and best practices play a pivotal role in maintaining ethical conduct in the digital landscape. As students and future coders, it is imperative to understand and abide by these laws to protect individual privacy. By implementing best practices such as informed consent, data minimization, encryption, software updates, and privacy-by-design, students can develop technology solutions that respect ethical principles and prioritize user privacy.

Ethical Implications of Data Breaches

In today's digital age, where technology permeates every aspect of our lives, the issue of data breaches has become a pressing concern. As students and future coders, it is crucial to understand the ethical implications of data breaches and the responsibility we hold in safeguarding sensitive information.

Data breaches occur when unauthorized individuals gain access to confidential data, such as personal information, financial records, or trade secrets, without the consent of the data owner. The consequences of these breaches can be devastating, both for individuals and organizations. Therefore, it is essential to delve into the ethical aspects surrounding data breaches to ensure we develop a strong ethical foundation as student coders.

First and foremost, one of the primary ethical implications of data breaches is the violation of privacy. Individuals have a right to privacy, and when their personal information is compromised, it infringes upon that right. As student coders, we must recognize the importance of protecting individuals' privacy and work towards developing secure systems that prevent unauthorized access to sensitive data.

Another ethical concern is the potential for identity theft and fraud. When personal information is stolen, it can be used maliciously, leading to financial loss and reputational damage. As ethical hackers, we need to understand the gravity of these consequences and ensure we design systems with robust security measures to mitigate the risk of data breaches.

Moreover, data breaches can also have far-reaching societal implications. Large-scale breaches can impact a significant number of people, eroding trust in digital systems and causing a sense of vulnerability. This erosion of trust can hinder technological advancements and impede the growth of digital economies. As student coders, it is our ethical duty to prioritize the security of our systems and contribute to building a trustworthy digital environment.

Lastly, data breaches may expose trade secrets and proprietary information, leading to financial losses for organizations. This can have a detrimental impact on innovation and competitiveness. As future coders, we must understand the ethical responsibility we bear in safeguarding organizations' intellectual property and contribute to creating secure systems that protect against such breaches.

In conclusion, the ethical implications of data breaches are multifaceted and should be taken seriously by students and future coders. Upholding the principles of privacy, security, and trust is essential in our roles as ethical hackers. By recognizing the importance of these ethical considerations, we can build a more secure and responsible digital landscape for the benefit of individuals, organizations, and society as a whole.

Chapter 5: Cybersecurity and Ethical Hacking

Cybersecurity Threat Landscape

In today's interconnected world, where technology plays a vital role in every aspect of our lives, the importance of cybersecurity cannot be emphasized enough. With the exponential growth of the internet and the increasing reliance on digital platforms, the threat landscape has become more complex and diverse than ever before. This subchapter will delve into the various aspects of the cybersecurity threat landscape, shedding light on the ethical challenges faced by student coders in this realm.

To truly understand the gravity of the situation, it is essential to comprehend the different types of cyber threats. From sophisticated hacking attempts to social engineering attacks, the threats posed by malicious actors can be overwhelming. The subchapter will explore the ethical implications associated with these threats, emphasizing the need for ethical hackers who can combat these dangers while maintaining a strong moral compass.

Students will gain insights into the motivations behind cyber attacks, ranging from financial gain to political agendas. By understanding these motives, they can better comprehend the ethical dilemmas that arise when attempting to protect individuals, organizations, and governments from cyber threats. The subchapter will encourage students to think critically about the ethical implications of their own coding practices and how their work can be exploited by cybercriminals.

Furthermore, the subchapter will highlight the importance of ethical considerations in cybersecurity. Students will learn about the legal and ethical frameworks that guide the actions of ethical hackers. They will explore the concept of responsible disclosure, understanding the balance between finding vulnerabilities and responsibly reporting them to ensure the safety of systems and users.

Importantly, the subchapter will emphasize the significance of ethical hacking as a legitimate profession. Students will gain an understanding of the ethical hacker's role in defending against cyber threats, not only in preventing attacks but also in identifying vulnerabilities and strengthening security measures. By examining real-world case studies, students will be able to grasp the tangible impact of ethical hacking on society.

In conclusion, the "Cybersecurity Threat Landscape" subchapter aims to provide students with a comprehensive understanding of the ever-evolving world of cyber threats. By exploring the ethical challenges faced by student coders, this subchapter encourages students to develop a strong ethical foundation to guide their coding practices. Ultimately, it aims to inspire the next generation of ethical hackers who will play a critical role in safeguarding digital systems and protecting individuals, organizations, and governments from the ever-present cybersecurity threats.

Ethical Hacking as a Cybersecurity Measure

In today's digital age, where technology plays a crucial role in our lives, ensuring the security of our data and systems has become more important than ever. Cybersecurity breaches have become a common occurrence, with malicious hackers constantly finding new ways to exploit vulnerabilities. To counter these threats, the field of ethical hacking has emerged as an effective cybersecurity measure.

Ethical hacking, also known as penetration testing or white-hat hacking, involves authorized individuals or teams simulating an attack on a computer system to identify its vulnerabilities. Unlike malicious hackers, ethical hackers operate within legal and ethical boundaries, with the sole purpose of enhancing security and preventing unauthorized access.

The primary goal of ethical hacking is to proactively identify weaknesses in a system before they can be exploited by malicious actors. By adopting the mindset of a hacker, ethical hackers can think like their adversaries and anticipate potential attack vectors. This approach allows organizations to patch vulnerabilities and strengthen their defenses before cybercriminals can exploit them.

Ethical hacking provides several key benefits to organizations and individuals. Firstly, it helps in identifying and addressing vulnerabilities that may have been overlooked during the development or implementation of a system. By conducting regular security audits, organizations can ensure that their systems are robust and resilient against potential threats.

Secondly, ethical hacking helps in staying one step ahead of cybercriminals. By constantly testing and assessing the security of a system, organizations can proactively identify emerging threats and take appropriate measures to mitigate them. This proactive approach is crucial in the ever-evolving landscape of cybersecurity, where new attack techniques and vulnerabilities are discovered regularly.

Moreover, ethical hacking promotes a culture of security-consciousness within organizations. By involving ethical hackers in the security process, organizations show their commitment to safeguarding sensitive data and protecting the privacy of their stakeholders.

However, it is important to understand the ethical implications of hacking. Ethical hackers must adhere to a strict code of conduct, respecting privacy and confidentiality. They should use their skills responsibly and only perform authorized penetration testing with proper consent. The ethical considerations of hacking are essential to ensure that the practice remains a positive force in cybersecurity.

In conclusion, ethical hacking has emerged as a vital cybersecurity measure in the face of increasing cyber threats. By adopting the mindset of hackers, ethical hackers help identify vulnerabilities, strengthen defenses, and stay ahead of malicious actors. However, it is crucial to approach hacking ethically and responsibly to maintain the trust and integrity of the cybersecurity community.

Addressing Cybersecurity Dilemmas Ethically

In today's interconnected world, the issue of cybersecurity has become a critical concern for individuals, organizations, and governments alike. As technology continues to advance rapidly, so do the threats posed by hackers and cybercriminals. It is essential for students, particularly those in the field of coding, to understand the ethical dilemmas that arise in the realm of cybersecurity and the importance of addressing them ethically.

Ethics play a significant role in guiding the decisions and actions of individuals, and the field of cybersecurity is no exception. As aspiring coders and technology enthusiasts, it is crucial to recognize the ethical implications of our work and the potential consequences it can have on others. This subchapter aims to shed light on some of the key ethical dilemmas faced by cybersecurity professionals and provide guidance on how to navigate them responsibly.

One of the most prominent ethical dilemmas in cybersecurity is the balance between privacy and security. As coders, we are often entrusted with developing tools and systems that protect sensitive information. However, it is important to consider the privacy rights of individuals and ensure that our actions do not infringe upon them. This dilemma requires us to find a balance between safeguarding against cyber threats and respecting individuals' right to privacy.

Another ethical dilemma is the responsibility of disclosing vulnerabilities. As ethical hackers, it is our duty to identify and report vulnerabilities in systems to prevent them from being exploited by malicious actors. However, this raises questions about responsible disclosure and the potential harm that can occur if vulnerabilities are made public before they can be adequately addressed. Finding the right balance between protecting users and informing system owners is crucial in this scenario.

Additionally, the ethical use of hacking tools and techniques is another dilemma that students must grapple with. While ethical hacking serves a noble purpose of identifying vulnerabilities and strengthening security measures, it is essential to use these tools responsibly and not engage in any malicious activities. Understanding the boundaries of ethical hacking and practicing it within legal and ethical limits is of utmost importance.

In conclusion, addressing cybersecurity dilemmas ethically is a critical aspect of being a responsible coder. As technology continues to evolve, so must our ethical considerations. By recognizing the ethical dilemmas in cybersecurity, such as the balance between privacy and security, responsible vulnerability disclosure, and ethical use of hacking tools, students can navigate these challenges responsibly. By doing so, we can contribute to a safer and more secure digital landscape while upholding the principles of ethics in our work.

Chapter 6: Ethical Hacking in Business and Society

The Role of Ethical Hacking in Business

In today's digital era, where businesses heavily rely on technology, the importance of ethical hacking cannot be overstated. Ethical hacking, also known as penetration testing or white-hat hacking, involves identifying vulnerabilities in a system or network to ensure its security. While hacking has negative connotations due to its association with malicious activities, ethical hacking serves a noble purpose – to protect businesses from potential cyber threats and breaches. This subchapter will delve into the pivotal role ethical hacking plays in the business world, enlightening student coders about the significance of ethical hacking in ensuring ethical practices and promoting a secure digital environment.

First and foremost, ethical hacking aids in identifying vulnerabilities in a company's network infrastructure. By conducting controlled attacks and exploiting weaknesses, ethical hackers can pinpoint potential entry points for cybercriminals. This information is invaluable for businesses as it allows them to patch these vulnerabilities before malicious hackers exploit them. Ethical hackers act as a safety net, ensuring that businesses are well-prepared to defend against cyber threats and safeguard their critical data.

Furthermore, ethical hacking is crucial for businesses to comply with ethical and legal standards. As technology advances, so do the regulations surrounding data privacy and cybersecurity. Companies need to stay up-to-date with these regulations to avoid legal consequences and reputational damage. Ethical hackers help businesses identify gaps in compliance and rectify them, ensuring that they meet the ethical standards set by regulatory bodies. This not only safeguards the company's reputation but also builds trust among customers, partners, and stakeholders.

Moreover, ethical hacking encourages businesses to adopt a proactive approach to security rather than a reactive one. By constantly testing and assessing their systems, companies can identify potential vulnerabilities before they are exploited. This proactive stance allows businesses to stay one step ahead of cybercriminals and minimize the potential impact of any breaches. Ethical hackers help create a culture of security awareness within organizations, where employees understand the importance of cybersecurity and actively work towards maintaining a secure environment.

In conclusion, ethical hacking plays a pivotal role in the business world by ensuring ethical practices, promoting cybersecurity, and protecting critical data. By identifying vulnerabilities, aiding compliance, and fostering a proactive security approach, ethical hackers contribute to a safer digital landscape. As student coders, it is essential to understand the ethical dimensions of hacking and recognize the significant role it plays in protecting businesses. By learning from ethical hacking practices, student coders can contribute to the development of secure and ethical technologies, making the digital world a safer place.

Ethical Hacking for Social Good

In today's increasingly connected world, where technology permeates every aspect of our lives, the need for ethical hackers has become more crucial than ever. Ethical hacking, also known as white-hat hacking, refers to the practice of using cybersecurity skills to identify and address vulnerabilities in computer systems and networks. While hacking is often associated with illegal activities and malicious intent, ethical hacking aims to ensure the security and integrity of digital infrastructure, making it an indispensable tool in the fight against cyber threats.

In this subchapter, we explore the concept of ethical hacking for social good, focusing on the ethical considerations and the positive impacts it can have on society. As students and future coders, it is essential to understand the ethical implications of our actions and how we can contribute to a safer digital environment.

Ethical hackers play a vital role in safeguarding individuals, organizations, and even nations from cyber threats. By proactively identifying vulnerabilities and weaknesses in systems, they help prevent potentially disastrous data breaches, financial losses, and privacy infringements. In doing so, they ensure that technology remains a force for good, enabling us to leverage its benefits without compromising our safety and well-being.

Moreover, ethical hacking promotes transparency and accountability in the digital realm. By exposing security flaws, ethical hackers not only help organizations patch vulnerabilities but also push for better cybersecurity practices and standards. This constant evaluation and improvement of systems contribute to the overall resilience of the digital infrastructure, making it increasingly difficult for malicious actors to exploit weaknesses.

However, ethical hacking must always be guided by a strong ethical framework. Students entering this field must understand the importance of obtaining proper authorization and informed consent before engaging in any hacking activities. Respecting privacy rights and maintaining confidentiality are crucial aspects of ethical hacking, ensuring that the line between ethical and illegal activities is not crossed.

Furthermore, ethical hackers must also be aware of the potential risks and unintended consequences of their actions. While their intentions may be noble, there is always a possibility of collateral damage or unintentional harm. Therefore, it is essential to exercise caution and responsibility when conducting security assessments and penetration testing.

In conclusion, ethical hacking for social good is a noble pursuit that combines technical expertise with a strong ethical foundation. As students and future coders, it is our responsibility to develop our skills in a manner that aligns with the principles of ethics and contributes positively to society. By understanding the ethical considerations involved in ethical hacking, we can harness our technical knowledge to make a meaningful impact, ensuring a safer and more secure digital future for all.

Ethical Challenges in Ethical Hacking Projects

In the exciting world of ethical hacking, where skilled individuals leverage their technical expertise for the greater good, there lie numerous ethical challenges that must be addressed. As aspiring ethical hackers, it is crucial for students to understand and navigate these challenges responsibly. This subchapter will delve into the ethical dilemmas faced by ethical hackers in their projects, offering insights and guidance on how to address them.

One of the primary ethical challenges in ethical hacking projects is the invasion of privacy. As ethical hackers, our goal is to identify vulnerabilities and potential threats in computer systems, networks, and software. However, this process often involves accessing sensitive information, which raises ethical concerns. Students must learn to strike a balance between obtaining necessary data for their projects and respecting the privacy of individuals and organizations. This entails obtaining proper consent and ensuring that data is handled securely and confidentially.

Another significant ethical challenge is the potential for unintended consequences. While ethical hackers aim to improve security, their actions can inadvertently cause harm. For instance, a vulnerability discovered during a project might be exploited by malicious actors before it can be patched. Students must approach their projects with caution, understanding that their actions can have far-reaching consequences. They should always prioritize responsible disclosure and work closely with organizations to mitigate any risks that may arise.

Furthermore, ethical hackers often face ethical dilemmas regarding the boundaries of their authorized access. It is essential for students to understand the terms of engagement and respect the limitations set by the organizations they are working with. Unauthorized access or exceeding the agreed-upon scope can lead to legal ramifications and damage the reputation of ethical hacking as a profession. Students should always seek proper authorization and maintain a clear line of communication with the organizations they are assisting.

Overall, ethical hacking projects present numerous ethical challenges that require careful consideration and adherence to ethical principles. As students interested in ethical hacking, it is crucial to prioritize ethics and responsible conduct in every step of the process. By respecting privacy, considering potential consequences, and adhering to authorized boundaries, ethical hackers can leverage their skills to make a positive impact on cybersecurity while upholding the highest ethical standards.

In conclusion, the ethical challenges posed by ethical hacking projects are complex and require careful thought. This subchapter aims to equip students with the knowledge and guidance needed to navigate these challenges responsibly. By understanding and addressing the ethical dilemmas that arise in ethical hacking projects, students can become ethical hackers who not only possess technical expertise but also demonstrate a strong commitment to ethical conduct and the highest standards of professionalism.

Chapter 7: Ethical Hacking and Intellectual Property

Intellectual Property Rights in Technology

In today's fast-paced world, where technology is advancing at an unprecedented rate, it is essential for student coders to understand the importance of intellectual property rights. As technology continues to shape our lives, the ethical implications surrounding the ownership and protection of ideas, innovations, and creations become increasingly relevant.

Intellectual Property (IP) refers to the legal rights granted to individuals or organizations for their original creations, inventions, or designs. In the realm of technology, IP encompasses a wide range of intangible assets, including software code, algorithms, patents, trademarks, and copyrights. As aspiring ethical hackers and student coders, it is crucial to respect and uphold these intellectual property rights.

One of the most fundamental aspects of intellectual property rights in technology is copyright protection. Copyright grants the creator of an original work exclusive rights to control its use and distribution. As students, it is essential to understand the importance of using software, code, or any digital content within the boundaries of copyright law. Plagiarism and unauthorized use of copyrighted materials not only harm the creators but also undermine the integrity of the coding community.

Another critical aspect of intellectual property rights in technology is patent protection. Patents provide inventors with exclusive rights to their inventions, preventing others from using, making, or selling the patented technology without permission. For students involved in technological innovation, understanding the patent system enables them to navigate the legal landscape and protect their own inventions from being exploited.

Trademarks also play a significant role in intellectual property rights. Trademarks are distinctive signs, symbols, or logos that identify and distinguish goods or services. As student coders, it is important to respect and avoid infringing upon established trademarks, as doing so can lead to legal consequences and damage the reputation of both individuals and companies.

In the realm of ethics, respecting intellectual property rights is not just a legal obligation but also a moral one. By honoring intellectual property rights, student coders foster a culture of innovation, fairness, and respect within the technology community. It allows creators to be rewarded for their efforts, encourages collaboration, and promotes the growth of new ideas.

In conclusion, intellectual property rights are a crucial aspect of technology ethics for student coders. By understanding and respecting copyright, patent, and trademark protection, students can contribute to a more ethical and sustainable technological landscape. Upholding these rights not only safeguards the interests of creators but also ensures the continued growth and progress of the coding community.

Ethical Hacking and Copyright Infringement

In today's digital age, the concept of hacking often conjures up images of cybercriminals bent on wreaking havoc and stealing sensitive information. However, not all hacking is malicious or unethical. Ethical hacking, also known as white-hat hacking, refers to the practice of identifying vulnerabilities in computer systems and networks to help organizations improve their security. While it is a noble pursuit, ethical hackers must navigate a complex landscape of legal and ethical considerations, particularly when it comes to copyright infringement.

Copyright infringement involves the unauthorized copying, distribution, or use of copyrighted material without the owner's permission. As students delving into the world of ethical hacking, it is crucial to understand the boundaries of copyright law and respect the rights of intellectual property owners.

Ethical hackers often encounter copyrighted software, documentation, or even proprietary code during their work. These materials are protected by copyright law, and reproducing or distributing them without explicit permission is illegal. It is imperative to remember that even with good intentions, violating copyright laws can have severe consequences, including legal action and damage to one's reputation.

To ensure ethical hacking practices, students should follow a set of guidelines when confronted with copyrighted material:

1. Obtain proper authorization: Before accessing any computer systems or networks, always seek explicit permission from the owner. This includes obtaining written consent to access and analyze any copyrighted material.

2. Limit usage: Use copyrighted material solely for the purpose of identifying vulnerabilities or improving security. Avoid any unnecessary reproduction, distribution, or use beyond what is required for ethical hacking activities.

3. Respect intellectual property: Do not share or distribute copyrighted material without proper authorization. Be mindful of the rights of intellectual property owners and their creative work.

4. Seek legal advice if unsure: If uncertain about the legality of using specific copyrighted material, consult legal professionals who can provide guidance on fair use, licensing, or other relevant copyright issues.

By adhering to these principles, student coders can ensure that their ethical hacking endeavors remain within the boundaries of copyright law. Respecting intellectual property not only upholds ethical standards but also helps foster a culture of trust and collaboration within the cybersecurity community.

Remember, ethical hacking is about improving security and protecting organizations from cyber threats. By staying informed, respecting copyrights, and always seeking proper authorization, student coders can contribute positively to the field of cybersecurity while maintaining the highest ethical standards.

Ethical Hacking and Patent Protection

In the ever-evolving world of technology, the concept of ethical hacking has gained significant attention. Ethical hackers, also known as white hat hackers, are individuals who use their skills to identify vulnerabilities in computer systems and networks, with the sole purpose of improving security measures. However, the intersection of ethical hacking and patent protection raises several ethical dilemmas that student coders need to be aware of.

Patent protection plays a crucial role in encouraging innovation by granting exclusive rights to inventors for their creations. It allows inventors to reap the benefits of their hard work and incentivizes further advancements. However, the challenge arises when ethical hackers discover vulnerabilities or weaknesses in patented technology.

One ethical dilemma is whether ethical hackers should disclose their findings to the patent holder or exploit the discovery for personal gain. As students interested in ethics, it is essential to understand the moral obligation to act in the best interest of society. In this case, it is crucial to prioritize the greater good over personal gain. By disclosing vulnerabilities to the patent holder, ethical hackers contribute to improving security and preventing potential harm to users.

Another ethical consideration is the potential conflict between patent protection and responsible disclosure. Patent holders may be reluctant to acknowledge vulnerabilities in their technology, fearing negative publicity or financial losses. However, responsible disclosure is vital for the overall security of the technology ecosystem. Student coders should understand the importance of responsible disclosure and the potential impact it can have on ensuring a safer digital environment.

Furthermore, ethical hackers should respect the intellectual property rights of patent holders. While they may identify vulnerabilities, they should refrain from unauthorized use or replication of patented technology. It is essential to strike a balance between ethical hacking and patent protection, ensuring that innovation is not hindered while safeguarding intellectual property rights.

To navigate these ethical dilemmas, it is crucial for students interested in ethical hacking to stay informed about patent laws and regulations. By understanding the legal framework, they can make informed decisions about responsible disclosure and how to contribute positively to the industry.

In conclusion, ethical hacking and patent protection intersect in complex ways, posing ethical dilemmas for student coders. By prioritizing the greater good, embracing responsible disclosure, and respecting intellectual property rights, students can navigate these dilemmas and contribute to a safer and more secure technology landscape.

Chapter 8: Ethical Hacking and Vulnerability Disclosure

Vulnerability Disclosure Ethics

In the rapidly evolving world of technology, ethical dilemmas are becoming increasingly common. One such dilemma that students entering the field of coding and technology must navigate is the issue of vulnerability disclosure ethics. As aspiring ethical hackers, it is crucial for students to understand the ethical considerations involved in discovering and disclosing vulnerabilities in software systems, websites, or networks.

Vulnerability disclosure refers to the practice of identifying and reporting security weaknesses in software or systems to the relevant parties, such as the software developers or system administrators. This process plays a crucial role in enhancing cybersecurity and preventing malicious attacks. However, it is essential to approach vulnerability disclosure with a clear set of ethics in mind.

First and foremost, students must understand the importance of responsible disclosure. When discovering a vulnerability, it may be tempting to exploit it or share it with others for personal gain. However, this goes against the principles of ethical hacking. Instead, responsible disclosure involves notifying the affected party about the vulnerability and giving them a reasonable amount of time to fix it before making it public. This allows the software developers or system administrators to address the issue and protect their users or systems from potential harm.

Moreover, students must consider the potential consequences of disclosing vulnerabilities. While the intention may be to improve security, disclosing vulnerabilities without proper consideration can lead to unintended negative consequences. For example, if a vulnerability is disclosed without giving the affected party enough time to fix it, malicious actors may exploit it before a patch can be implemented, causing significant harm. Therefore, students must carefully weigh the potential benefits and risks before disclosing a vulnerability.

Additionally, students should be aware of the legal and ethical implications of vulnerability disclosure. Different countries and regions may have specific laws surrounding the disclosure of vulnerabilities, and violating these laws can have serious consequences. It is essential to research and understand the legal landscape and adhere to ethical guidelines when disclosing vulnerabilities.

Lastly, students must also consider the ethical responsibility to educate and empower others. Sharing knowledge and best practices regarding vulnerability disclosure can help improve overall cybersecurity. By educating software developers and system administrators on how to identify and fix vulnerabilities, students can contribute to a more secure digital environment.

In conclusion, vulnerability disclosure ethics is a crucial topic for students entering the field of coding and technology. Responsible disclosure, consideration of consequences, adherence to legal and ethical guidelines, and a commitment to education are key components of ethical vulnerability disclosure. By understanding and practicing these principles, students can become ethical hackers who contribute to a safer and more secure digital world.

Responsible Disclosure Programs

In an increasingly interconnected world, the role of ethical hackers and their contribution to cybersecurity has become more crucial than ever. As student coders, it is essential to understand the importance of responsible disclosure programs and how they can help maintain a secure digital landscape. This subchapter will explore the significance of responsible disclosure programs and their ethical implications.

Responsible disclosure programs, also known as bug bounty programs or vulnerability disclosure programs, are initiatives created by organizations to encourage ethical hackers to report security vulnerabilities they discover in their systems. These programs establish a framework for ethical hackers to responsibly disclose any loopholes or weaknesses they find, allowing the organization to address the issue before it can be exploited by malicious actors.

One of the primary reasons responsible disclosure programs are crucial is that they promote a collaborative and transparent approach to cybersecurity. By incentivizing ethical hackers to report vulnerabilities, organizations create a mutually beneficial relationship. Ethical hackers gain recognition, monetary rewards, or even job opportunities, while organizations can identify and fix vulnerabilities before they can be exploited. This cooperative effort helps maintain the integrity and security of digital systems.

Additionally, responsible disclosure programs align with ethical principles by emphasizing the importance of privacy, data protection, and user safety. By reporting vulnerabilities to organizations rather than exploiting them for personal gain, ethical hackers demonstrate their commitment to responsible and ethical behavior. This approach ensures that users' personal information remains secure, minimizing the risk of data breaches and potential harm.

However, it is crucial for students to understand the ethical considerations associated with responsible disclosure programs. Ethical hackers must adhere to guidelines set by organizations and respect their boundaries. It is essential to act responsibly, maintain confidentiality, and not engage in any unauthorized actions beyond identifying and reporting vulnerabilities.

Moreover, responsible disclosure programs also raise questions about the balance between ethical hacking and the legal framework surrounding it. Students need to be aware of the laws and regulations governing hacking activities in their respective jurisdictions. Engaging in hacking activities without proper authorization can have severe legal consequences, even if the intention is ethical.

In conclusion, responsible disclosure programs are a vital component of the cybersecurity landscape. For student coders interested in ethics, it is crucial to recognize the benefits of these programs in maintaining a secure digital environment. By participating in responsible disclosure programs, ethical hackers can contribute to the protection of user data, privacy, and overall system security. However, it is equally important to understand and abide by the ethical guidelines and legal boundaries associated with these programs.

The Ethical Hacker's Role in Vulnerability Management

In the ever-evolving world of technology, the need for ethical hackers has become increasingly significant. With the rise of cyber threats and vulnerabilities, organizations are seeking skilled professionals who can identify and address security loopholes before malicious hackers exploit them. This subchapter explores the crucial role of ethical hackers in vulnerability management, shedding light on their ethical responsibilities and the impact they have on ensuring the integrity of digital systems.

Ethical hackers, also known as white hat hackers, are individuals who use their skills and knowledge to identify and rectify security vulnerabilities in computer systems. They work with organizations to conduct penetration testing, vulnerability assessments, and risk analysis to proactively identify potential weaknesses in software, networks, or applications. By adopting the mindset of a malicious hacker, ethical hackers can anticipate and mitigate potential threats.

One of the primary ethical responsibilities of an ethical hacker is to ensure that their actions are legal and authorized. They must obtain written consent from the organization before conducting any security testing or assessments. Additionally, ethical hackers must use their skills solely for the purpose of identifying vulnerabilities, without causing harm or stealing sensitive information. Their goal is to help organizations strengthen their security measures, protect user data, and prevent potential cyber-attacks.

Vulnerability management is a critical aspect of an organization's cybersecurity strategy. Ethical hackers play a vital role in this process by identifying vulnerabilities and providing recommendations for remediation. They leverage their expertise to simulate real-world attack scenarios, testing the resilience of systems and infrastructure. Through their efforts, ethical hackers can help organizations stay one step ahead of potential cyber threats, ensuring that their systems are secure and resilient to attacks.

For students interested in the field of ethical hacking, it is essential to understand the ethical implications associated with vulnerability management. While the work of an ethical hacker may seem exciting and challenging, it comes with a great deal of responsibility. Students must prioritize ethics and adhere to legal guidelines to ensure they are making a positive impact in the field.

In conclusion, the role of ethical hackers in vulnerability management is critical in today's digital landscape. By identifying and addressing security vulnerabilities, ethical hackers help organizations fortify their defenses against potential cyber-attacks. However, it is important for students to recognize the ethical considerations that come with this role, ensuring that their actions are lawful and in alignment with their ethical responsibilities. By embracing these principles, students can become valuable assets in the fight against cybercrime while upholding the highest standards of ethics.

Chapter 9: Ethical Hacking and Social Engineering

Understanding Social Engineering Tactics

In the digital age, where technology has become an integral part of our lives, it is crucial to be aware of the various threats that lurk in the virtual world. While advancements in technology have brought numerous benefits, they have also given rise to an array of malicious activities, one of which is social engineering. This subchapter aims to provide students with a comprehensive understanding of social engineering tactics and their ethical implications.

Social engineering is the art of manipulating individuals to divulge sensitive information or perform specific actions that could potentially compromise their privacy or security. These tactics exploit human psychology, taking advantage of trust, fear, and curiosity. It often involves impersonation, deception, or manipulation to gain unauthorized access to systems, networks, or personal data.

Ethical hackers, also known as white hat hackers, employ social engineering techniques to identify vulnerabilities in systems and raise awareness about potential risks. By understanding how social engineering works, students can learn to protect themselves and others from falling victim to such attacks.

One common social engineering tactic is phishing, where attackers trick individuals into revealing their personal information or login credentials through fraudulent emails or websites. Students must be cautious and verify the authenticity of such requests before sharing any sensitive information online.

Another tactic is pretexting, where an attacker creates a compelling scenario to gain the trust of their target. For example, they might pose as a reputable organization or a trusted individual to extract information. Students should be skeptical of unsolicited communications and always verify the identity of the person or organization before sharing confidential information.

Understanding the motivations behind social engineering attacks is essential for ethical hackers. Some attackers aim to gain unauthorized access to systems for financial gain, while others might seek personal information for identity theft or corporate espionage. Students must recognize the ethical implications of such actions and understand the importance of respecting privacy and security.

By studying social engineering tactics, students can develop a heightened sense of skepticism, critical thinking, and digital resilience. They will be better equipped to protect themselves and others from falling victim to social engineering attacks. Additionally, ethical hackers can use this knowledge to educate others about the risks and promote responsible online behavior.

In conclusion, understanding social engineering tactics is crucial in today's digital world. By being aware of the various tactics employed by malicious actors, students can enhance their ethical hacking skills, protect themselves from potential threats, and contribute to building a safer online environment.

Ethical Implications of Social Engineering

In today's interconnected world, technology plays a pivotal role in our daily lives. As students and future coders, it is essential to not only understand the technical aspects of our field but also the ethical implications that arise from our actions. One such area that requires careful consideration is social engineering.

Social engineering refers to the manipulation of human psychology to gain unauthorized access to sensitive information or systems. It involves exploiting human trust, curiosity, and vulnerabilities rather than relying solely on technical vulnerabilities. While social engineering techniques can be used for legitimate purposes, it often becomes a tool for malicious intent.

The ethical implications of social engineering are profound and multifaceted. Firstly, it raises concerns about privacy invasion and the potential misuse of personal data. Social engineering attacks can lead to the unauthorized access of personal information, financial data, or even control over someone's online identity. As ethical hackers, it is our responsibility to protect individuals' privacy and ensure that their personal information remains secure.

Secondly, social engineering attacks can have severe consequences on individuals and organizations. By exploiting human trust, attackers can manipulate people into divulging sensitive information or performing actions that could harm themselves or their organization. As student coders, we have the responsibility to build robust systems that are resistant to such attacks, safeguarding the interests of individuals and organizations alike.

Furthermore, the ethical implications extend beyond individuals and organizations to society as a whole. Social engineering attacks can undermine public trust in technology and erode confidence in online interactions. This can have far-reaching consequences, such as decreased adoption of digital services or increased skepticism towards online platforms. As future coders, it is our duty to promote a secure and trustworthy digital environment.

To address these ethical implications, it is crucial for students to be well-versed in social engineering techniques. By understanding the methods used by attackers, we can develop better defenses and educate others about potential risks. Additionally, ethical hackers play a vital role in identifying vulnerabilities and helping organizations build resilient systems.

In conclusion, the ethical implications of social engineering demand our attention as student coders. We must recognize the potential harm caused by social engineering attacks and take proactive steps to mitigate them. By prioritizing privacy, security, and trust, we can contribute to a safer and more ethical technological landscape for everyone.

Ethical Hacking to Combat Social Engineering Attacks

In today's interconnected world, where technology plays a pivotal role in our daily lives, the threat of cyberattacks and data breaches has become a pressing concern. As students and future coders, it is essential to not only understand the intricacies of technology but also to recognize the ethical dilemmas associated with it. One such dilemma revolves around the practice of ethical hacking, particularly in combating social engineering attacks.

Social engineering attacks are a type of cyber threat where hackers manipulate individuals through psychological manipulation to gain unauthorized access to sensitive information or systems. These attacks exploit human vulnerabilities rather than technical flaws, making them a significant challenge to detect and prevent. However, ethical hacking can be a powerful tool in combating these attacks while adhering to ethical principles.

Ethical hackers, also known as white-hat hackers, use their skills and knowledge to identify and rectify vulnerabilities within an organization's systems. In the context of social engineering attacks, ethical hackers employ various techniques to assess an organization's susceptibility to manipulation and devise countermeasures to protect against such attacks.

One approach ethical hackers use is called phishing simulations. By creating simulated phishing emails or messages, they test an organization's employees' ability to recognize and respond appropriately to potential threats. These simulations serve as eye-opening experiences for individuals, enhancing their awareness and alertness towards social engineering attacks.

Another technique employed by ethical hackers is the use of social engineering audits. These audits involve analyzing an organization's policies and procedures to identify potential weaknesses that could be exploited by malicious actors. Ethical hackers then recommend necessary changes and improvements to mitigate the risks associated with social engineering attacks.

It is crucial for students to understand that ethical hacking, when conducted within legal and moral boundaries, can be a valuable tool in ensuring the security and privacy of individuals and organizations. By studying and practicing ethical hacking techniques, students can develop a deep understanding of the potential vulnerabilities that social engineering attacks exploit and contribute to the development of robust security measures.

However, it is equally important to remember the ethical aspect of ethical hacking. Students must always obtain proper authorization and use their skills responsibly, ensuring that their actions do not cause harm or intrude on individuals' privacy. Upholding ethical standards is paramount in the field of ethical hacking and helps distinguish it from malicious hacking activities.

In conclusion, ethical hacking can be a powerful means to combat social engineering attacks. Through techniques such as phishing simulations and social engineering audits, ethical hackers can assess vulnerabilities, educate individuals, and strengthen an organization's security posture. As students, it is essential to approach ethical hacking with a strong sense of ethics and responsibility, contributing to a safer and more secure digital landscape for all.

Chapter 10: Ethical Hacking and Future Technology

Emerging Technologies and Ethical Concerns

In today's rapidly evolving digital landscape, emerging technologies have the potential to revolutionize the way we live, work, and interact with the world around us. From artificial intelligence and blockchain to virtual reality and the Internet of Things, these technologies hold immense promise for innovation and progress. However, as students and aspiring coders, it is essential to recognize and address the ethical concerns that arise with their implementation.

One of the primary ethical concerns surrounding emerging technologies is privacy. With the increasing amount of data being collected and analyzed, there is a growing need to protect individuals' personal information. As students, it is crucial to understand the importance of data security and privacy, as well as the potential consequences of mishandling or misusing sensitive information.

Another significant concern is the potential impact of emerging technologies on employment and the job market. While these technologies have the potential to automate and streamline various processes, they also raise questions about job displacement and the need for retraining or upskilling. As students, it is essential to consider the ethical implications of technology adoption and ensure that our creations do not contribute to societal inequalities.

Furthermore, ethical concerns related to bias and discrimination cannot be overlooked. Artificial intelligence, for instance, heavily relies on data to make informed decisions. However, if the data used to train

AI algorithms is biased or discriminatory, it can perpetuate existing inequalities and reinforce systemic biases. As students, it is crucial to develop AI systems that are fair, transparent, and accountable, mitigating the risks of bias and discrimination.

Additionally, emerging technologies can pose significant challenges when it comes to cybersecurity and protecting against malicious actors. As coders, we must ensure that the systems we build are secure and resilient, keeping in mind potential vulnerabilities and the potential harm that can be caused by cyberattacks.

In conclusion, while emerging technologies offer countless possibilities for innovation and progress, it is important for students and aspiring coders to understand and address the ethical concerns that accompany their development and implementation. By actively considering privacy, employment, bias, discrimination, and cybersecurity, we can create a future that is not only technologically advanced but also ethically sound. As ethical hackers, it is our responsibility to unravel technology dilemmas and ensure that the benefits of emerging technologies are enjoyed by all, with integrity and fairness.

Ethical Hacking in Artificial Intelligence

In recent years, the rapid advancement of artificial intelligence (AI) has revolutionized various industries and transformed the way we live and interact with technology. From smart homes and autonomous vehicles to virtual assistants and personalized recommendations, AI has become an integral part of our daily lives. However, with this increased reliance on AI comes the need for ethical considerations, particularly in the field of hacking.

Ethical hacking, also known as white-hat hacking, refers to the practice of identifying vulnerabilities and weaknesses in computer systems and networks with the permission of the owner, in order to improve their security. It involves using the same techniques and tools as malicious hackers, but with the intention of preventing cyber-attacks and safeguarding sensitive information.

When it comes to AI, ethical hacking plays a crucial role in ensuring the security and integrity of these sophisticated systems. AI algorithms are designed to learn from data and make decisions based on patterns and trends. However, they are not immune to vulnerabilities and can be exploited by malicious actors to manipulate or compromise their functionality.

By applying ethical hacking principles, students interested in AI and ethics can contribute to the development of secure and trustworthy AI systems. They can help identify potential vulnerabilities in AI algorithms, assess the robustness of AI models against adversarial attacks, and propose countermeasures to mitigate these risks.

One of the key ethical dilemmas in AI is the issue of bias. AI algorithms are trained on large datasets, which may contain biased information, leading to biased outcomes. Ethical hackers can play a vital role in identifying and rectifying these biases, ensuring that AI systems are fair and unbiased.

Moreover, ethical hacking can also contribute to the protection of personal privacy and data security. As AI systems collect vast amounts of user data, it is essential to ensure that this data is appropriately protected. Ethical hackers can help organizations identify and address potential vulnerabilities in AI systems that could lead to data breaches or privacy violations.

In conclusion, ethical hacking in artificial intelligence is a critical aspect of ensuring the security, fairness, and trustworthiness of AI systems. Students interested in ethics and AI have the opportunity to make a positive impact by applying ethical hacking principles to identify and mitigate vulnerabilities in AI algorithms. By doing so, they can contribute to the development of ethical and responsible AI, making the world a safer place for everyone.

Ethical Considerations for Future Technology Developers

In today's rapidly advancing world, technology has become an integral part of our lives. As students and aspiring technology developers, it is crucial to understand the ethical considerations that come with creating and implementing new technologies. In this subchapter, we will explore the key ethical principles that future technology developers should keep in mind.

First and foremost, it is essential to prioritize the well-being and safety of individuals and society as a whole. As technology developers, we have a responsibility to ensure that our creations do not cause harm or infringe upon the rights of others. This means considering potential risks and taking steps to mitigate them. For example, when developing artificial intelligence systems, we must ensure that they are not biased or discriminatory.

Transparency and accountability are also vital ethical considerations. It is important to be open and honest about the capabilities and limitations of our technologies. Users should have a clear understanding of how their data is collected, stored, and used. Additionally, as developers, we should be accountable for any unintended consequences that arise from our creations. This means being responsive to feedback, addressing vulnerabilities, and continuously improving our technology.

Respecting privacy and promoting data security are crucial aspects of ethical technology development. Students must understand the importance of obtaining informed consent when collecting personal data. It is also essential to implement robust security measures to protect user information from unauthorized access or misuse. By respecting privacy rights and ensuring data security, we can build trust with users and foster a more ethical technological landscape.

Another ethical consideration is inclusivity and accessibility. Technology should be designed with the needs and preferences of a diverse range of users in mind. This means considering factors such as age, gender, disability, and cultural background. By creating inclusive technologies, we can ensure that everyone has equal access and opportunities.

Lastly, ethical technology development involves staying up-to-date with legal and regulatory frameworks. As students, it is essential to be aware of laws and regulations pertaining to technology and data. By complying with these laws, we can ensure that our creations are ethically sound and contribute positively to society.

In conclusion, future technology developers must be mindful of the ethical considerations surrounding their work. By prioritizing the well-being of individuals, being transparent and accountable, respecting privacy and promoting data security, embracing inclusivity and accessibility, and staying informed about legal and regulatory frameworks, students can become ethical technology developers who contribute to a better and more responsible technological future.

Chapter 11: Conclusion

Recap of Ethical Hacking Principles

In this subchapter, we will revisit the fundamental principles of ethical hacking that we have discussed thus far. As students delving into the world of ethical hacking, it is essential to understand the principles that guide our actions and ensure we stay on the right path. Ethics play a crucial role in this field, as they help us maintain integrity, respect, and responsibility while exploring the realm of technology.

1. Permission and Consent:
Ethical hackers must always obtain proper permission and consent before engaging in any hacking activities. This means seeking authorization from the system owner or administrator to test their security measures. Without explicit permission, any hacking attempts are considered unethical and illegal.

2. Intent:
The intent behind ethical hacking is to identify vulnerabilities and weaknesses in systems with the aim of improving their security. It is crucial to remember that the goal is not to cause harm, steal data, or disrupt operations. Our actions should always align with the purpose of enhancing security and preventing potential cyber threats.

3. Confidentiality:
Respecting confidentiality is a fundamental principle in ethical hacking. Any information obtained during the hacking process should be handled with care and kept confidential. Sharing sensitive data

without proper authorization is a breach of ethical standards and can have severe consequences.

4. Responsiveness:
Ethical hackers must promptly report any vulnerabilities discovered to the system owners or administrators. Timely communication allows for necessary actions to be taken to address the identified issues, preventing potential cyber attacks. Responsiveness is a key aspect of ethical hacking, as it helps maintain trust and strengthens security measures.

5. Continuous Learning:
The field of ethical hacking is constantly evolving, with new vulnerabilities and technologies emerging regularly. As students, it is vital to recognize the importance of continuous learning and staying updated with the latest techniques and security protocols. This will enable us to adapt and respond effectively to ever-changing cyber threats.

By adhering to these ethical hacking principles, we can ensure that our actions remain within the boundaries of legality and morality. As students exploring the field of ethical hacking, it is our responsibility to uphold these principles and use our knowledge to protect and secure systems rather than exploit them. With a strong foundation in ethics, we can become responsible and respected professionals in the realm of technology, making a positive impact on the cybersecurity landscape.

The Importance of Ethical Hacking for Student Coders

In today's digital age, where technology is an integral part of our daily lives, it is crucial for student coders to understand the significance of ethical hacking. As technology continues to advance rapidly, so do the potential risks and vulnerabilities that can be exploited by malicious individuals. Hence, a strong foundation in ethical hacking is not only essential for students pursuing careers in cybersecurity but also for every student coder.

Ethical hacking, also known as penetration testing or white-hat hacking, involves identifying vulnerabilities in computer systems, networks, and software applications. Unlike malicious hackers, ethical hackers use their skills and knowledge to protect and secure these systems from potential threats. They play a pivotal role in ensuring the safety of sensitive information, safeguarding personal privacy, and maintaining the integrity of digital infrastructure.

For student coders, understanding ethical hacking is crucial for several reasons. Firstly, it provides them with a unique perspective on the vulnerabilities that exist within the systems they develop. By adopting an ethical hacker's mindset, student coders can proactively identify and address security flaws during the development process, making their software more robust and less susceptible to cyberattacks. This not only enhances their reputation as skilled coders but also contributes to the overall security of digital systems.

Secondly, ethical hacking instills a strong sense of ethics and responsibility among student coders. It emphasizes the importance of respecting privacy, adhering to legal and ethical standards, and using their skills for the greater good. By understanding the ethical implications of hacking and learning how to navigate complex ethical dilemmas, student coders can make informed decisions and contribute positively to the digital world.

Furthermore, ethical hacking opens up numerous career opportunities for student coders. With the increasing demand for cybersecurity experts, companies are actively seeking individuals with a strong ethical hacking background. By acquiring these skills, students can position themselves as valuable assets in the job market and embark on exciting and fulfilling cybersecurity careers.

In conclusion, ethical hacking plays a pivotal role in the lives of student coders. It equips them with valuable knowledge, skills, and ethical considerations necessary to navigate the evolving technological landscape. By understanding the importance of ethical hacking, student coders can contribute to creating a safer digital world, enhance their career prospects, and become responsible digital citizens.

Ethical Hacking as a Career Path for Ethical Coders

Introduction:

In today's digital age, where technology governs almost every aspect of our lives, the need for ethical coders has never been greater. With the increasing number of cyber threats and the vulnerability of our online systems, it has become crucial to have professionals who possess the skills to protect our digital world. One such career path that combines ethical coding skills with an ethical mindset is that of an ethical hacker. This subchapter will explore the exciting world of ethical hacking and how it can be a rewarding career choice for students with a strong ethical foundation.

Understanding Ethical Hacking:

Ethical hacking, also known as penetration testing or white-hat hacking, involves identifying vulnerabilities in computer systems, networks, and software applications. Unlike malicious hackers, ethical hackers use their skills to discover weaknesses and suggest improvements, ultimately enhancing the security of these systems. They work closely with organizations to strengthen their defenses against potential cyberattacks, ensuring the protection of sensitive data and maintaining the integrity of digital infrastructures.

The Role of Ethical Coders in Ethical Hacking:

Ethical hacking heavily relies on the knowledge and expertise of ethical coders. These individuals possess a deep understanding of programming languages, software development, and system architectures. Their ability to analyze code, identify vulnerabilities, and develop secure solutions is crucial in the ethical hacking process. Ethical coders bring a unique perspective to the table, as they not only have the technical skills but also a deep understanding of ethical principles and the importance of protecting user privacy.

Ethics in Ethical Hacking:

Ethics play a fundamental role in the field of ethical hacking. Ethical hackers must abide by a strict code of conduct, ensuring that they operate within legal boundaries and respect the privacy rights of individuals and organizations. They must obtain proper authorization before conducting any penetration testing and handle sensitive information responsibly. Ethical coders, with their strong ethical foundation, are well-equipped to navigate the complex ethical dilemmas that may arise in this field.

Career Opportunities:

The demand for ethical hackers is on the rise, as organizations recognize the importance of securing their digital assets. Ethical coders with a passion for cybersecurity and an ethical mindset have a plethora of career opportunities in this field. They can work in various sectors, including government agencies, financial institutions, technology companies, and consulting firms. Moreover, ethical hackers can also choose to work independently as freelance consultants, providing their expertise to organizations on a project basis.

Conclusion:

Ethical hacking offers a promising career path for students with a strong ethical foundation and coding skills. As technology continues to evolve, the need for ethical coders who can protect our digital infrastructure becomes increasingly critical. By pursuing a career in ethical hacking, students can combine their passion for coding with their ethical principles, making a positive impact on the cybersecurity landscape while contributing to a safer digital world.

Printed by Libri Plureos GmbH in Hamburg, Germany